UNDERSTANDING AMYOTROPHIC LATERAL SCLEROSIS

Comprehensive Guide To Symptoms, Diagnosis, Treatment Options, And Management Strategies For Patients

DR. LINCOLN WAYLON

DISCLAIMER

This book contains information that should only be used for educational and informational reasons; it is not meant to be used as a source of medical or psychological advice. The author's studies, life experiences, and expertise in the area of health and wellness served as the foundation for the content. It should not, however, be used in place of expert counsel, a diagnosis, or medical care.

Any queries you may have about a physical or mental health issue should always be directed toward the advice of a licensed healthcare provider or mental health specialist. With regard to the efficacy or outcomes of the methods or suggestions included in this book, the author and publisher make no representations or warranties.

Any information or methods in this book are used entirely at the reader's own risk and discretion. The material provided here may be used or misused, and neither the author nor the publisher will be held responsible for any results, losses, or negative impacts.

Keep in mind that everyone has different demands and reactions to health and wellness routines. Any health and wellness plans you implement must be customized to your particular circumstances, and you should speak with experts to make sure the plans meet your needs.

TABLE OF CONTENTS

ABOUT THE BOOK

"Understanding Amyotrophic Lateral Sclerosis" serves as an essential guide for individuals seeking comprehensive insights into ALS, a condition that profoundly impacts both patients and their families. This book provides a thorough overview of Amyotrophic Lateral Sclerosis, beginning with a clear definition and a historical context that frames the condition's evolution over time.

It offers crucial statistics and prevalence data, distinguishing ALS from other similar neurological disorders, and emphasizes the significant effects the disease has on daily living. Understanding these foundational aspects is critical for anyone affected by ALS or involved in care and support.

The book delves into the causes and risk factors associated with ALS, exploring both established theories and ongoing research. It examines genetic factors and heredity, environmental risks, and lifestyle considerations, providing a nuanced understanding of what may contribute to the onset of this disease. By highlighting current research efforts, the book sheds light on the future directions of ALS studies, offering hope and clarity about potential breakthroughs.

Symptoms of ALS are discussed in detail, from early signs to the progression of motor and non-motor symptoms. The book outlines how these symptoms impact physical and cognitive functions, noting the variability among patients. This section is crucial for recognizing and understanding the disease's trajectory and how it manifests differently in each individual.

Diagnostic processes are thoroughly explained, including the criteria and guidelines used by healthcare professionals. The role of neurologists in diagnosing ALS and differentiating it from other conditions is emphasized, along with the importance of early diagnosis for effective management and treatment.

Current treatment options and management strategies are presented, covering available medications, non-pharmacological therapies, and supportive care such as physical therapy and nutritional support. The role of multidisciplinary care teams in providing comprehensive care is highlighted, showcasing how coordinated efforts can enhance patient outcomes.

Living with ALS is addressed with practical advice on managing daily activities and accessing emotional and psychological support. The book offers guidance on adaptive equipment and technologies, support networks, and coping strategies, ensuring that both patients and their families are equipped with the tools needed for daily life.

The section on ALS research and advances provides an overview of recent breakthroughs, emerging treatments, and the role of genetics and biotechnology in shaping future therapies. It encourages readers to engage with ongoing research and stay informed about potential new treatments.

Legal and financial considerations are discussed, offering information on legal rights, financial planning, insurance coverage, and workplace accommodations. This section aims to assist individuals in navigating the practical challenges that arise with ALS.

Support systems and resources are comprehensively covered, including support groups, online forums, professional counseling, and community resources. The book provides a wealth of information on accessing and utilizing these resources to ensure ongoing support and education.

Detailed FAQs address common concerns such as the early symptoms of ALS, diagnostic procedures, available treatments, support groups, and future research prospects. This section offers quick, accessible answers to frequently asked questions, making it a valuable reference for those seeking immediate information.

CHAPTER ONE

OVERVIEW OF AMYOTROPHIC LATERAL SCLEROSIS

DEFINITION AND GENERAL INFORMATION

Amyotrophic Lateral Sclerosis (ALS) is a progressive neurodegenerative disorder that primarily affects the motor neurons in the brain and spinal cord. This condition leads to muscle weakness, loss of motor control, and eventual paralysis. ALS, often referred to as Lou Gehrig's disease, disrupts the communication between the brain and muscles, making it increasingly difficult for individuals to perform basic voluntary movements. As the disease advances, it progressively impairs the ability to speak, swallow, and breathe, with many patients eventually requiring full-time care.

ALS is characterized by the degeneration of both upper and lower motor neurons. The upper motor neurons, which are located in the brain, and the lower motor neurons, which extend from the spinal cord to the muscles, both become progressively damaged. This results in symptoms such as muscle cramping, stiffness, and twitching, followed by muscle weakness and atrophy. Despite affecting motor functions, ALS does not typically impair cognitive abilities, though some patients may experience changes in behavior or thinking.

Early symptoms of ALS often include difficulty with fine motor skills and muscle cramps or twitches. As the disease progresses, individuals may experience challenges with walking, speaking, and swallowing. The exact cause of ALS remains unknown, but genetic and environmental factors are believed to play a role in its development. There is currently no cure, and treatment focuses on managing symptoms and improving quality of life.

HISTORICAL BACKGROUND OF ALS

The history of Amyotrophic Lateral Sclerosis dates back to the late 19th century when the condition was first described by French neurologist Jean-Martin

Charcot. Charcot, who is considered the father of neurology, identified the disease's distinct symptoms and coined the term "Amyotrophic Lateral Sclerosis" to describe the condition. His pioneering work laid the groundwork for future research and helped establish ALS as a distinct clinical entity.

The disease gained broader public recognition in the 20th century, largely due to the high-profile case of baseball player Lou Gehrig. Gehrig, diagnosed with ALS in 1939, brought significant attention to the condition through his public battle and poignant farewell speech. This increased awareness led to heightened research efforts and the establishment of various ALS associations and support networks aimed at improving patient care and advancing scientific understanding.

Over the years, significant progress has been made in ALS research, including the discovery of genetic mutations linked to familial forms of the disease. The establishment of dedicated research centers and collaborations among scientists, clinicians, and patients has facilitated advances in both understanding the disease's pathology and developing potential treatments. Despite these efforts, ALS remains a challenging and incurable condition.

KEY STATISTICS AND PREVALENCE

Amyotrophic Lateral Sclerosis is relatively rare, with an estimated prevalence of 4-7 cases per 100,000 people worldwide. In the United States, approximately 16,000 individuals are living with ALS, with about 5,000 new diagnoses occurring each year. The incidence of ALS generally increases with age, with most cases being diagnosed between the ages of 40 and 70.

Geographical variation in ALS prevalence has been observed, with higher rates reported in some regions compared to others. For instance, studies have shown increased incidence in certain countries, such as the United States and France, while lower rates are observed in other parts of the world. Research into these variations continues, as understanding the factors contributing to regional differences may help in identifying potential environmental or genetic influences.

ALS affects both men and women, though men are slightly more likely to be diagnosed with the disease. The lifetime risk of developing ALS is approximately 1 in 400, with variations based on genetic predisposition and environmental factors. Efforts to track and record ALS statistics are crucial for understanding the disease's impact and guiding public health initiatives and research priorities.

DIFFERENTIATION FROM SIMILAR CONDITIONS

Amyotrophic Lateral Sclerosis can be challenging to differentiate from other neurodegenerative conditions due to overlapping symptoms. Unlike Multiple Sclerosis (MS), which primarily affects the central nervous system with episodes of relapse and remission, ALS is characterized by a gradual, continuous decline in motor function without periods of improvement.

The presence of both upper and lower motor neuron signs helps distinguish ALS from conditions like Parkinson's disease, which predominantly affects movement control without the widespread muscle atrophy seen in ALS.

Another condition that can be confused with ALS is Spinal Muscular Atrophy (SMA), a genetic disorder that also causes muscle weakness and atrophy. However, SMA typically presents in childhood and is associated with different genetic mutations compared to ALS. Furthermore, ALS does not usually include the significant sensory loss seen in conditions such as Peripheral Neuropathy, which affects the peripheral nerves and can cause pain and numbness.

Correct diagnosis of ALS often requires a comprehensive neurological examination and the exclusion of other diseases with similar presentations. Advanced imaging techniques, electromyography

(EMG), and lumbar puncture can help confirm the diagnosis by identifying characteristic patterns of motor neuron damage and ruling out other possible conditions. Accurate differentiation is essential for appropriate treatment and management.

THE IMPACT ON DAILY LIFE

Amyotrophic Lateral Sclerosis profoundly affects daily life as the disease progresses. Initially, individuals may experience mild symptoms such as difficulty with fine motor tasks or slight muscle weakness, but these issues can quickly escalate to more severe impairments. As muscle strength declines, basic activities such as dressing, eating, and mobility become increasingly challenging, often necessitating adaptations or the use of assistive devices.

The impact on communication and swallowing can significantly affect quality of life. Many individuals with ALS experience speech difficulties due to weakened muscles, leading to the need for speech-generating devices or alternative communication methods. Similarly, difficulties with swallowing can pose risks for malnutrition and aspiration, often requiring dietary modifications or feeding tubes to ensure adequate nutrition.

Emotional and psychological challenges are also prevalent among individuals with ALS and their families. The progressive nature of the disease, combined with the loss of independence and increasing dependence on caregivers, can lead to feelings of frustration, depression, and anxiety. Support from healthcare professionals, counseling, and support groups play a crucial role in helping individuals and families navigate these challenges and maintain quality of life throughout the disease's progression.

CHAPTER TWO

CAUSES AND RISK FACTORS

KNOWN CAUSES AND THEORIES

Amyotrophic Lateral Sclerosis (ALS) remains an enigmatic condition, with its exact causes still not fully understood. However, researchers have identified several key theories that offer insight into the potential origins of the disease. One prominent theory is that ALS results from a combination of genetic mutations and environmental factors. Studies have revealed that certain genetic mutations, such as those in the SOD1 gene, are linked to familial forms of ALS, which account for a small percentage of cases. In contrast, sporadic ALS, which represents the majority of cases, does not have a clear genetic marker but may be influenced by complex interactions between genes and environmental triggers.

The role of oxidative stress is another crucial theory. This involves damage to cells caused by free radicals, which are unstable molecules that can harm cellular structures.

In ALS, oxidative stress may contribute to the degeneration of motor neurons, leading to the progressive muscle weakness characteristic of the disease. Researchers are also exploring the role of protein misfolding, where abnormal proteins accumulate in motor neurons, disrupting their function and leading to cell death. This understanding is crucial in developing targeted treatments and interventions.

The theory of autoimmune response is yet another area of investigation. Some scientists propose that ALS may result from the body's immune system mistakenly attacking its motor neurons. This theory is supported by the presence of inflammatory cells in the spinal cord and brain of ALS patients. While these theories provide valuable insights, the precise mechanisms underlying ALS continue to be a subject of active research, to uncover more about how the disease develops and progresses.

GENETIC FACTORS AND HEREDITY

Genetic factors play a significant role in the development of Amyotrophic Lateral Sclerosis, particularly in familial cases where the condition is inherited. Approximately 5-10% of ALS cases are familial, meaning they occur in families with a history of the disease. Mutations in specific genes, such as SOD1, C9orf72, and TARDBP, have been identified as contributing to these inherited forms of ALS. Understanding these genetic factors is essential for early diagnosis and family planning, as genetic testing can identify individuals at risk and offer guidance on preventive measures or monitoring.

In familial ALS, the inheritance pattern can be autosomal dominant, meaning a single copy of the mutated gene from one parent is enough to increase the risk of developing the disease. This contrasts with sporadic ALS, where no clear inheritance pattern is observed. Genetic research has focused on uncovering the specific mutations responsible for these familial cases and understanding how they lead to motor neuron degeneration.

This research also aims to identify potential targets for gene-based therapies that could halt or slow the progression of the disease.

Genetic counseling is an important aspect for families affected by ALS. It helps individuals understand their risk of developing or passing on the disease and provides information on available testing options. Counseling can also assist in making informed decisions about family planning and participating in clinical trials aimed at finding effective treatments or preventive strategies. By advancing our knowledge of genetic factors, researchers are working towards more personalized approaches to ALS treatment and management.

ENVIRONMENTAL RISK FACTORS

Environmental factors are believed to contribute to the development of Amyotrophic Lateral Sclerosis, although the exact mechanisms remain unclear. Studies have explored various environmental exposures, such as pesticides, heavy metals, and industrial chemicals, as potential risk factors. For instance, agricultural workers who are regularly exposed to pesticides have shown a slightly higher risk of developing ALS. This has led to investigations into how such chemicals might influence the disease process, possibly through mechanisms like oxidative stress or neuroinflammation.

Another area of interest is the potential link between physical trauma and ALS. Research has examined whether repeated head injuries or strenuous physical activity might increase the risk of developing the disease. Some studies suggest that athletes, especially those involved in contact sports, may have a higher incidence of ALS, prompting further investigation into how physical stress might impact motor neuron health. The exact relationship remains under study, but these findings highlight the need for further research into environmental influences on ALS risk.

The complexity of environmental factors lies in their interactions with genetic predispositions. ALS likely results from a combination of genetic susceptibility and exposure to environmental triggers.

 This interaction is challenging to study but is crucial for understanding how external factors contribute to the onset and progression of ALS. Ongoing research aims to clarify these connections and identify modifiable environmental risk factors that could be targeted to prevent or reduce the impact of ALS.

LIFESTYLE CONSIDERATIONS

Lifestyle factors have been investigated as potential contributors to the risk of developing Amyotrophic Lateral Sclerosis. Diet, exercise, and overall health may play roles in the disease's onset and progression.

For example, some research has explored the impact of dietary choices, such as high-fat or low-antioxidant diets, on ALS risk. While evidence is still emerging, maintaining a balanced diet rich in antioxidants and omega-3 fatty acids may offer protective benefits and support overall motor neuron health.

Physical activity and exercise are also under scrutiny, with studies examining whether regular physical activity might influence ALS risk. Although there is no conclusive evidence linking exercise directly to ALS prevention or progression, staying physically active is generally beneficial for overall health and may help manage some symptoms of the disease. Conversely, excessive physical strain or repetitive stress might be harmful, emphasizing the need for balanced and moderated exercise routines.

Smoking and alcohol consumption are lifestyle factors that have been studied for their potential effects on ALS. Smoking is known to contribute to a range of health issues, including neurodegenerative diseases, while excessive alcohol consumption can lead to neurological damage. Reducing or eliminating these risk factors is advisable for overall health and may contribute to lowering the risk of developing ALS.

Adopting a healthy lifestyle, including avoiding smoking and excessive drinking, maybe a proactive measure for reducing ALS risks.

ONGOING RESEARCH ON CAUSES

Ongoing research into the causes of Amyotrophic Lateral Sclerosis is focused on unraveling the complex interplay of genetic, environmental, and biological factors that contribute to the disease. Scientists are investigating new genetic mutations and their roles in ALS, aiming to discover additional biomarkers that could aid in early diagnosis and treatment. Advances in genomic technology and bioinformatics are enabling researchers to identify novel gene-environment interactions that could provide new insights into the disease's etiology.

Researchers are also exploring the role of cellular and molecular mechanisms in ALS. This includes studying how abnormal protein aggregation, mitochondrial dysfunction, and neuroinflammation contribute to motor neuron degeneration.

Innovative techniques such as stem cell research and advanced imaging are being used to model ALS and test potential therapies. These studies are crucial for developing targeted treatments that address the underlying mechanisms of the disease.

Clinical trials are an essential component of ongoing ALS research, providing opportunities to test new drugs and interventions. Researchers are evaluating various approaches, from gene therapy and drug repurposing to lifestyle interventions and supportive therapies. The goal is to identify effective treatments that can slow or halt the progression of ALS and ultimately improve the quality of life for patients. Continued investment in research and collaboration across scientific disciplines are key to making progress in understanding and combating ALS.

CHAPTER THREE

SYMPTOMS OF ALS

EARLY SIGNS AND SYMPTOMS

Amyotrophic Lateral Sclerosis (ALS) often begins subtly, making it challenging to pinpoint. Early signs may include muscle twitching or weakness, typically starting in one part of the body, such as the hands or legs. Individuals might notice difficulty in performing fine motor tasks, like buttoning a shirt or typing, which can be mistaken for common age-related changes or stress.

As the disease progresses, muscle weakness become more pronounced, leading to a noticeable decrease in strength and dexterity.

Patients might struggle with walking or balancing, experiencing frequent trips or falls. Difficulty in speaking clearly or swallowing food can also become apparent, signaling the onset of more serious symptoms.

At this stage, recognizing these early signs is crucial for diagnosis and management. The subtle changes in muscle function, combined with difficulty in daily tasks, should prompt a consultation with a healthcare provider to evaluate symptoms and initiate diagnostic tests.

PROGRESSION OF SYMPTOMS

As ALS advances, the initial localized symptoms spread to other muscle groups, resulting in broader functional impairments. Muscle weakness and atrophy become more generalized, affecting the arms, legs, and trunk. This progression often leads to severe mobility issues, requiring the use of mobility aids like wheelchairs or walkers for assistance.

The progression also impacts speech and swallowing muscles, causing further difficulties in communication and eating. Patients may develop dysarthria, characterized by slurred or slow speech, and dysphagia, making it challenging to swallow liquids and solids. These symptoms necessitate dietary modifications and potentially the use of feeding tubes.

The progression rate can vary among individuals, but the overall impact on daily activities and independence increases significantly. Regular monitoring and adjustments in care strategies are essential to manage the evolving symptoms and maintain quality of life.

MOTOR AND NON-MOTOR SYMPTOMS

Motor symptoms in ALS primarily involve muscle weakness and atrophy, affecting voluntary movements and coordination. This includes difficulty with tasks requiring precise movements, like writing or lifting objects, and may lead to muscle cramps and spasms. The gradual loss of muscle strength impacts both upper and lower limbs, resulting in reduced mobility and functionality.

Non-motor symptoms, while less visible, play a significant role in the disease's progression.

These may include emotional changes such as depression or anxiety, often linked to the challenges of living with a progressive illness.

Cognitive changes, including difficulties with memory or executive functions, can also occur, impacting daily living and mental health.

Addressing both motor and non-motor symptoms requires a comprehensive approach, including physical therapy to manage motor impairments and psychological support to handle emotional and cognitive changes. This holistic care strategy helps improve overall well-being and functionality.

DIFFERENCES IN SYMPTOMS AMONG PATIENTS

ALS presents with a wide spectrum of symptoms, and the disease's manifestation can vary greatly from one individual to another. Some patients may experience an early onset of limb weakness, while others may have initial difficulties with speech or swallowing.

The rate of symptom progression and the specific muscles affected also differ, leading to a unique disease trajectory for each person.

Variability in symptoms can impact the choice of treatment and management strategies. Personalized care plans, tailored to address the specific symptoms and progression rate of each patient, are crucial for effective disease management. Regular assessments and adjustments to the care approach ensure that treatment aligns with the individual's evolving needs.

Understanding these differences helps in providing targeted support and interventions. By recognizing and addressing the specific symptoms and progression patterns, healthcare providers can offer more effective management strategies and improve the quality of life for each patient.

IMPACT ON PHYSICAL AND COGNITIVE FUNCTIONS

ALS has a profound impact on both physical and cognitive functions, affecting daily living and overall quality of life. Physically, the disease causes progressive muscle weakness, leading to difficulties with movement, balance, and coordination. Patients may experience increased fatigue and require assistive devices for mobility and daily activities.

Cognitively, while many patients retain their intellectual abilities, some may experience changes in memory, problem-solving, and executive functions. These cognitive impairments can affect daily decision-making and social interactions, adding another layer of complexity to the disease's management.

The combined impact on physical and cognitive functions necessitates a multidisciplinary approach to care, including physical therapy for motor symptoms and cognitive support for mental challenges. This comprehensive care helps in managing the disease's multifaceted effects and supporting patients in maintaining their independence and quality of life.

CHAPTER FOUR

DIAGNOSIS OF ALS

DIAGNOSTIC CRITERIA AND GUIDELINES

Amyotrophic lateral sclerosis (ALS) diagnosis follows specific criteria outlined by various medical guidelines, primarily focusing on identifying the disease through clinical presentation and neurological examination. The most recognized criteria are provided by the El Escorial criteria and the revised Airlie House criteria, which emphasize the presence of both upper and lower motor neuron signs in multiple regions of the body. This involves documenting symptoms such as muscle weakness, atrophy, and spasticity, alongside ruling out other conditions with similar presentations. For a definitive diagnosis, clinicians typically require evidence of progressive muscle weakness and a combination of both upper and lower motor neuron involvement, without any other neurological disease explaining these findings.

The guidelines also stress the importance of ruling out other diseases through a comprehensive assessment of the patient's medical history, clinical symptoms, and family history. This process includes evaluating the onset and progression of symptoms to ensure they align with the characteristic pattern of ALS. The diagnostic criteria aim to ensure that ALS is not mistaken for other neurological conditions with overlapping symptoms, such as multiple sclerosis or progressive muscular atrophy. Accurate adherence to these criteria is essential for proper diagnosis and subsequent management of the disease.

Clinicians may use specific diagnostic guidelines, such as those from the American Academy of Neurology (AAN) or the World Federation of Neurology (WFN), which provide detailed frameworks for diagnosing ALS. These guidelines help standardize the diagnostic process, ensuring consistency across different medical settings. By following these established criteria, healthcare professionals can systematically evaluate and diagnose ALS, contributing to more effective treatment planning and patient care.

DIAGNOSTIC TESTS AND PROCEDURES

The diagnosis of ALS often involves a combination of tests and procedures designed to assess motor function and exclude other possible conditions. One of the primary diagnostic tools is electromyography (EMG), which measures electrical activity in muscles to detect signs of motor neuron damage. EMG can identify abnormal muscle electrical activity that is characteristic of ALS, such as denervation and reinnervation patterns. Additionally, nerve conduction studies are used to evaluate the speed and strength of nerve impulses, helping to rule out peripheral neuropathies that might mimic ALS symptoms.

Magnetic Resonance Imaging (MRI) is another crucial diagnostic procedure, used to visualize the spinal cord and brain to identify any structural abnormalities or lesions that could suggest other neurological disorders. Although MRI is not diagnostic for ALS per se, it helps exclude other conditions such as tumors or herniated discs that could present with similar symptoms. Additionally, blood tests and cerebrospinal fluid (CSF) analysis may be performed to rule out infectious or inflammatory causes of muscle weakness and to evaluate overall neurological health.

Genetic testing is increasingly used to identify familial forms of ALS and can be particularly useful if there is a known family history of the disease. This testing can help confirm the diagnosis when genetic mutations associated with ALS are found. By combining these diagnostic tests and procedures, clinicians can achieve a more accurate diagnosis, ensuring that ALS is correctly identified and managed based on the individual patient's condition.

ROLE OF NEUROLOGISTS IN DIAGNOSIS

Neurologists play a central role in diagnosing ALS, leveraging their expertise in neuromuscular disorders to interpret clinical symptoms and diagnostic test results. Their involvement begins with a thorough neurological examination, where they assess muscle strength, coordination, reflexes, and other motor functions. Neurologists are skilled in distinguishing ALS from other conditions that may present with similar symptoms, such as Parkinson's disease or peripheral neuropathy, through detailed patient history and examination.

In addition to conducting physical assessments, neurologists are responsible for coordinating diagnostic tests and interpreting their results. They utilize their knowledge of various diagnostic criteria and guidelines to evaluate EMG findings, MRI results, and other diagnostic data. Neurologists also play a key role in consulting with other specialists when necessary, ensuring a comprehensive approach to diagnosis and ruling out other potential causes of the patient's symptoms.

Furthermore, neurologists are involved in discussing the diagnosis with patients and their families, providing information about the disease, its progression, and potential treatment options. They offer guidance on managing symptoms and navigating the emotional and practical aspects of living with ALS. By guiding patients through the diagnostic process and offering support, neurologists ensure that patients receive accurate diagnoses and appropriate care.

DIFFERENTIAL DIAGNOSIS PROCESS

The differential diagnosis process for ALS involves systematically ruling out other conditions that can present with similar symptoms, ensuring an accurate diagnosis. This process begins with a detailed patient history and physical examination to identify the specific nature of the symptoms and their progression.

Conditions that are commonly differentiated from ALS include multiple sclerosis, which may present with similar motor symptoms but typically involves relapsing and remitting episodes, and spinal muscular atrophy, which often has a different age of onset and progression pattern.

Diagnostic tests play a crucial role in the differential diagnosis process. For example, imaging studies like MRI can help differentiate ALS from conditions that involve structural abnormalities of the brain or spinal cord. Blood tests and cerebrospinal fluid analysis are also used to rule out infections, autoimmune diseases, and metabolic disorders that could mimic ALS symptoms. Genetic testing can further assist in distinguishing familial ALS from other hereditary neuromuscular disorders.

The differential diagnosis process requires careful consideration of the patient's clinical presentation and response to treatment. By evaluating the progression of symptoms, response to therapies, and results of diagnostic tests, healthcare providers can narrow down the list of potential diagnoses. This thorough approach ensures that ALS is accurately identified and other conditions are appropriately managed or excluded.

IMPORTANCE OF EARLY DIAGNOSIS

Early diagnosis of ALS is crucial for optimizing patient outcomes and managing the disease effectively. Identifying ALS in its early stages allows for timely intervention, which can help slow disease progression and improve quality of life. Early diagnosis enables patients to begin treatments that may help manage symptoms and potentially extend functional abilities.

It also allows for early involvement in clinical trials and access to experimental therapies that could offer additional benefits.

Moreover, an early diagnosis provides patients and their families with valuable time to plan for the future. This includes making decisions about care, treatment options, and potential lifestyle adjustments. Early diagnosis also allows for early referral to multidisciplinary care teams, which can offer comprehensive support in managing the physical, emotional, and practical challenges associated with ALS.

From a healthcare perspective, early diagnosis can lead to more efficient use of resources and better coordination of care. It allows for a proactive approach to managing symptoms and complications, potentially reducing hospitalizations and improving overall patient outcomes. By emphasizing the importance of early diagnosis, healthcare professionals can help ensure that patients receive timely and effective care.

CHAPTER FIVE

CURRENT TREATMENTS AND MANAGEMENT

AVAILABLE MEDICATIONS AND THEIR EFFECTS

The treatment of Amyotrophic Lateral Sclerosis (ALS) involves a range of medications designed to manage symptoms and potentially slow disease progression. Riluzole, a commonly prescribed drug, is known to extend survival and time before tracheostomy by reducing glutamate levels in the brain, which can help slow neuron damage. Another medication, Edaravone, has been shown to reduce oxidative stress and may help in slowing functional decline. These drugs are often used in combination with other therapies to maximize patient benefits.

Medications like Baclofen or Tizanidine are used to address spasticity, a common symptom in ALS patients, helping to alleviate muscle stiffness and improve movement. For managing pain, neuropathic pain medications such as Gabapentin or Pregabalin may be prescribed. Additionally, medications to manage excessive saliva, such as Glycopyrrolate, can help improve comfort and quality of life for those affected by bulbar symptoms.

Regular monitoring and adjustment of medication regimens are crucial, as ALS symptoms and responses to treatment can change over time. Patients should maintain ongoing communication with their healthcare providers to ensure that any side effects or new symptoms are addressed promptly, and medication effectiveness is optimized.

NON-PHARMACOLOGICAL TREATMENTS

Non-pharmacological treatments for ALS focus on improving quality of life and managing symptoms without the use of drugs. Occupational therapy is vital in helping patients maintain their independence and perform daily activities more efficiently. Therapists can recommend adaptive equipment, such as modified utensils or wheelchairs, to assist with mobility and daily tasks.

Speech therapy plays a significant role in managing bulbar symptoms, such as difficulties with speaking and swallowing. Therapists can provide techniques to enhance communication and suggest communication devices if necessary.

Swallowing difficulties can be managed through dietary modifications and strategies to minimize choking risk.

Cognitive behavioral therapy and counseling can also be beneficial in addressing the emotional and psychological challenges that come with ALS. These therapies help patients and families cope with the stress and emotional impact of the disease, providing strategies for mental and emotional support.

PHYSICAL THERAPY AND REHABILITATION

Physical therapy is essential in managing the physical aspects of ALS, helping to maintain mobility and function as long as possible. Therapists design individualized exercise programs to improve strength, flexibility, and endurance, focusing on low-impact exercises that reduce the risk of injury and overexertion.

Rehabilitation efforts often include range-of-motion exercises to prevent joint contractures and muscle atrophy. Assistive devices, such as braces or orthotic supports, may be used to enhance mobility and provide stability.

Regular physical therapy sessions can help in managing fatigue and maintaining an optimal level of physical activity, which is crucial in slowing the progression of physical decline. Collaboration with a multidisciplinary team ensures that rehabilitation efforts are coordinated with other aspects of ALS management for comprehensive care.

NUTRITIONAL AND RESPIRATORY SUPPORT

Proper nutritional support is crucial for ALS patients to maintain strength and overall health. Dietitians work with patients to develop meal plans that meet their specific needs, addressing issues such as dysphagia (difficulty swallowing) by recommending texture-modified diets or feeding tubes if necessary. Nutritional supplements may be prescribed to ensure adequate caloric and nutrient intake.

Respiratory support becomes increasingly important as ALS progresses, due to the weakening of respiratory muscles. Non-invasive ventilation options, such as bi-level-positive airway pressure (BiPAP), can assist with breathing during sleep and help manage daytime respiratory difficulties. In advanced cases, invasive ventilation methods, including tracheostomy, may be considered.

Regular monitoring of respiratory function and timely intervention are essential in managing complications related to breathing. Coordination with respiratory therapists ensures that appropriate measures are taken to maintain optimal lung function and address any issues related to respiratory support.

ROLE OF MULTIDISCIPLINARY CARE TEAMS

Multidisciplinary care teams are integral to the comprehensive management of ALS, providing a coordinated approach to address the complex needs of patients. These teams typically include neurologists, physical therapists, occupational therapists, speech therapists, dietitians, and respiratory therapists, each contributing specialized expertise to the patient's care.

Regular team meetings and communication ensure that all aspects of the patient's condition are addressed, and treatment plans are adjusted as needed. This collaborative approach helps in managing symptoms effectively, improving patient outcomes, and ensuring that care is tailored to the individual's needs.

Engaging with a multidisciplinary team also facilitates access to additional resources and support services, such as social workers and counselors.

CHAPTER SIX

LIVING WITH ALS

MANAGING DAILY LIFE AND ACTIVITIES

Living with Amyotrophic Lateral Sclerosis (ALS) involves adapting daily routines to accommodate physical limitations that increase over time. For individuals managing ALS, it is crucial to establish a structured routine that emphasizes safety and independence. This might involve modifying the home environment to reduce hazards, such as installing grab bars in bathrooms and using non-slip mats on floors. Activities such as meal preparation can be streamlined using adaptive tools, like utensils with larger grips or pre-prepared meals to minimize effort and ensure nutritional needs are met.

Daily activities, from dressing to personal hygiene, may require adaptive strategies and tools. Clothing with Velcro fastenings instead of buttons or zippers can make dressing easier, while shower chairs and handheld shower heads can assist with bathing. It is beneficial to plan and prioritize tasks to conserve energy and reduce fatigue, breaking activities into smaller, manageable steps and incorporating rest periods throughout the day. By customizing the approach to daily life, individuals with ALS can maintain a degree of independence and comfort.

Implementing home modifications and using adaptive technologies can also enhance quality of life. Voice-activated devices or smart home systems can help with managing lights, thermostats, and entertainment systems, minimizing physical effort. It is essential to regularly review and adjust these adaptations as the condition progresses to ensure they continue to meet changing needs effectively.

EMOTIONAL AND PSYCHOLOGICAL SUPPORT

Living with ALS presents significant emotional and psychological challenges for both patients and their families. Providing a supportive environment involves acknowledging and addressing feelings of fear, frustration, and grief. Mental health professionals, such as counselors or psychologists with experience in chronic illness, can offer valuable support by helping individuals and families navigate the emotional aspects of the disease, developing coping strategies, and addressing mental health concerns.

Support groups, either in-person or online, can offer a sense of community and shared experience. These groups allow individuals with ALS and their families to connect with others facing similar challenges, share personal stories, and gain insights into coping strategies. Engaging in these communities can provide comfort and reduce feelings of isolation, fostering a network of emotional support.

Encouraging open communication within the family is also crucial. Families should make space for discussing fears, hopes, and expectations openly. Regular conversations can help in understanding each other's emotional needs and making adjustments to support each other effectively. Maintaining strong family bonds and addressing emotional needs proactively can greatly enhance overall well-being.

ADAPTIVE EQUIPMENT AND TECHNOLOGIES

Adaptive equipment and technologies play a pivotal role in managing the daily challenges of ALS. Devices such as powered wheelchairs, mobility aids, and custom seating can enhance physical mobility and comfort. For tasks requiring fine motor skills, specialized tools like modified keyboards and touch screens with larger icons can help maintain communication and computer use. It is essential to consult with occupational therapists or assistive technology specialists to select and customize equipment that best suits individual needs.

Communication devices, including speech-generating devices and eye-tracking technology, are vital for those experiencing significant speech difficulties. These technologies enable users to communicate more effectively, providing a means to interact with others and express their needs and thoughts. Regular assessments by professionals can ensure that the technology used remains effective as the condition evolves.

Maintaining and upgrading adaptive equipment is also important for ensuring ongoing functionality and comfort. Regular check-ups and adjustments to equipment can prevent complications and accommodate any changes in physical abilities. By integrating these technologies and equipment into daily life, individuals with ALS can enhance their independence and quality of life.

SUPPORT NETWORKS AND RESOURCES

Support networks and resources are crucial for navigating the complexities of living with ALS.

Connecting with local ALS associations or organizations can provide access to resources such as financial assistance, home care services, and educational materials. These organizations often offer workshops, support groups, and advocacy services that can aid in managing the disease and accessing necessary care.

Building a support network involving healthcare providers, social workers, and community organizations can offer comprehensive assistance. Healthcare providers can help with medical management, while social workers can assist with coordinating care and navigating insurance or financial concerns. Community resources, including volunteer services and local charities, may also provide practical support, such as transportation or respite care.

Engaging with online forums and social media groups dedicated to ALS can also be beneficial. These platforms provide a space for sharing experiences, seeking advice, and finding emotional support from a global community. By leveraging these networks and resources, individuals with ALS and their families can gain valuable information and support tailored to their needs.

COPING STRATEGIES FOR PATIENTS AND FAMILIES

Coping with ALS requires developing strategies to manage the physical, emotional, and logistical aspects of the disease. For patients, adopting a proactive approach to managing symptoms and maintaining physical health is essential. This might involve working with healthcare providers to create a personalized care plan, incorporating physical therapy to maintain mobility, and using relaxation techniques to manage stress and pain.

Families also need to develop coping strategies to handle the demands of caregiving and maintain their well-being. Establishing a support system, including seeking help from friends, family members, or professional caregivers, can alleviate the burden of caregiving responsibilities. Families need to schedule regular breaks and engage in self-care activities to prevent burnout and maintain a healthy balance.

Education and open communication are key components in coping effectively.

Families should stay informed about ALS and its progression to make informed decisions about care and support. Open discussions about roles, expectations, and concerns can help in managing the evolving needs of the patient while maintaining family harmony and emotional health.

CHAPTER SEVEN

ALS RESEARCH AND ADVANCES
OVERVIEW OF RECENT RESEARCH BREAKTHROUGHS

Recent research breakthroughs in Amyotrophic Lateral Sclerosis (ALS) have significantly advanced our understanding of the disease. Cutting-edge studies have identified new biomarkers that enable earlier detection of ALS, potentially leading to more effective interventions. One notable breakthrough is the discovery of genetic mutations associated with familial ALS, which has opened new pathways for targeted therapies. Researchers have also made progress in understanding the role of glial cells in disease progression, revealing potential new drug targets that could slow down or even halt the disease.

These advancements are supported by innovative technologies such as high-throughput sequencing and advanced imaging techniques. High-throughput sequencing allows scientists to analyze vast amounts of genetic data rapidly, identifying mutations and variations that contribute to ALS. Advanced imaging techniques provide detailed insights into the progression of ALS at a cellular level, enhancing our ability to monitor disease progression and response to treatment.

The integration of these breakthroughs into clinical practice is paving the way for more personalized and effective treatment approaches. By understanding the molecular and cellular mechanisms underlying ALS, researchers are developing targeted therapies that address the specific needs of individual patients. This personalized approach holds promise for improving outcomes and extending the quality of life for those affected by ALS.

EMERGING TREATMENTS AND CLINICAL TRIALS

Emerging treatments for ALS are at the forefront of clinical research, offering hope for more effective management of the disease. One promising approach is gene therapy, which aims to correct or replace defective genes responsible for ALS. Clinical trials are exploring the potential of gene-editing technologies, such as CRISPR, to target and modify genetic mutations associated with the disease. These trials are still in the early stages but show great promise in providing a long-term solution for patients.

Additionally, stem cell therapy is being investigated as a means to repair damaged motor neurons and slow disease progression. Researchers are testing various types of stem cells, including neural stem cells and induced pluripotent stem cells, to determine their effectiveness in treating ALS. Clinical trials are focusing on the safety and efficacy of these therapies, to develop treatments that can regenerate damaged tissues and restore motor function.

Another area of active research is the development of new drugs that target specific pathways involved in ALS. These drugs aim to reduce neuroinflammation, protect motor neurons, and improve overall muscle function. Ongoing clinical trials are assessing the safety and effectiveness of these novel compounds, providing hope for new treatment options that could significantly impact the management of ALS.

THE ROLE OF GENETICS AND BIOTECHNOLOGY

Genetics and biotechnology play a crucial role in advancing our understanding of ALS and developing new treatments. Recent genetic studies have identified several genes associated with both familial and sporadic forms of ALS. This genetic insight has led to the development of targeted therapies that aim to address specific genetic mutations. Biotechnology tools, such as RNA interference and gene editing, are being employed to modify or suppress these mutations, potentially providing a cure for genetic forms of ALS.

Biotechnology also contributes to the development of diagnostic tools and therapeutic strategies. Techniques such as next-generation sequencing enable the detailed analysis of genetic variants, helping researchers identify potential drug targets and biomarkers.

Additionally, biotechnology advancements are facilitating the creation of animal models that mimic human ALS, allowing scientists to test new treatments and gain insights into disease mechanisms.

The integration of genetic and biotechnological approaches into ALS research is accelerating the development of personalized medicine. By tailoring treatments based on an individual's genetic profile, researchers aim to enhance the effectiveness of therapies and improve patient outcomes. This precision medicine approach holds the potential to revolutionize ALS treatment and provide more targeted and effective solutions.

IMPACT OF RESEARCH ON FUTURE TREATMENTS

Research into ALS is driving significant advancements in future treatments, with ongoing studies promising to transform the management of the disease. The identification of new biomarkers and disease mechanisms is paving the way for earlier diagnosis and more precise targeting of therapies. This progress is expected to lead to the development of treatments that not only slow disease progression but also address the underlying causes of ALS.

The integration of innovative technologies, such as gene editing and stem cell therapy, into research is likely to yield breakthroughs in treatment options. These technologies offer the potential to repair or replace damaged motor neurons and correct genetic mutations, providing hope for more effective and long-lasting therapies. As research continues to evolve, the focus on personalized medicine and targeted therapies is expected to improve the quality of life for ALS patients.

Moreover, the collaborative efforts between researchers, clinicians, and patients are enhancing the translation of research findings into clinical practice. Increased funding and support for ALS research are contributing to the rapid advancement of new treatments and ensuring that promising discoveries reach that in need.

The continued focus on research and innovation will be crucial in shaping the future of ALS treatment and improving patient outcomes.

HOW TO GET INVOLVED IN RESEARCH

Getting involved in ALS research offers an opportunity to contribute to the advancement of treatments and support those affected by the disease. One way to participate is by volunteering for clinical trials, which provide access to new therapies and help researchers evaluate their effectiveness. Clinical trial registries and research centers often seek volunteers with ALS or healthy individuals for various studies, and participating in these trials can have a significant impact on the development of new treatments.

Another avenue for involvement is through advocacy and fundraising efforts. Supporting organizations dedicated to ALS research and awareness can help drive funding for innovative projects and support ongoing research initiatives. By participating in fundraising events, spreading awareness, and advocating for increased research funding, individuals can contribute to the progress of ALS research and help bring new treatments to those in need.

Additionally, staying informed about ongoing research and developments in ALS can provide opportunities to get involved in community-based research initiatives. Many research institutions and organizations offer educational programs and workshops that allow individuals to learn more about ALS and participate in research-related activities. Engaging with these opportunities can help individuals stay connected with the latest advancements and contribute to the collective effort to find a cure for ALS.

CHAPTER EIGHT

LEGAL AND FINANCIAL CONSIDERATIONS

LEGAL RIGHTS AND ADVOCACY

Understanding the legal rights and advocacy options available to individuals with Amyotrophic Lateral Sclerosis (ALS) is crucial for navigating the challenges of the disease. Advocacy groups and legal organizations offer resources and support to ensure that people with ALS are informed about their rights and have access to necessary services.

These organizations often guide navigating disability benefits, legal protections under the Americans with Disabilities Act (ADA), and other relevant laws designed to safeguard individuals with disabilities.

Legal rights include the right to access accommodations in public spaces and workplaces, as well as protection against discrimination. Advocacy efforts focus on raising awareness about ALS and influencing policy changes to improve access to medical care and support services. Engaging with these organizations can help individuals with ALS and their families understand their rights, access legal assistance, and advocate for necessary changes in policies and services.

Effective advocacy often involves connecting with local or national ALS support groups, legal aid organizations, or disability rights advocates. These groups can assist with filing complaints, applying for benefits, and ensuring that individuals receive the support they are legally entitled to. Staying informed and actively participating in advocacy can empower individuals with ALS to navigate their legal rights more effectively.

FINANCIAL PLANNING AND ASSISTANCE

Financial planning for individuals with ALS requires careful consideration of the costs associated with medical care, assistive devices, and daily living expenses. A comprehensive financial plan should include budgeting for ongoing medical treatments, potential modifications to the home, and other expenses that may arise as the disease progresses. Consulting with a financial advisor who has experience working with individuals with chronic illnesses can provide valuable insights into managing these costs.

There are various financial assistance programs available to support individuals with ALS. These may include government benefits such as Social Security Disability Insurance (SSDI) and Supplemental Security Income (SSI), as well as state and local programs that offer grants or subsidies for medical and home care expenses. It is important to research and apply for these programs early to ensure timely access to financial support.

In addition to public assistance programs, exploring options such as private insurance policies and charitable organizations can help cover costs not fully addressed by government programs. Keeping track of all financial resources and regularly reviewing the financial plan can help manage expenses and ensure that sufficient funds are available to meet ongoing needs.

INSURANCE AND HEALTHCARE COVERAGE

Navigating insurance and healthcare coverage is a key aspect of managing ALS. It is essential to understand what your health insurance plan covers, including treatments, medications, and specialized care. Review your policy to determine the extent of coverage for ALS-related expenses and identify any potential gaps. Contacting insurance providers to clarify coverage details and explore options for additional or supplemental insurance can help ensure that you have the necessary support.

Many individuals with ALS may qualify for government-sponsored healthcare programs such as Medicaid or Medicare, which can offer additional support for medical expenses. These programs have specific eligibility requirements and coverage options, so it is important to understand how they can complement your existing insurance.

Applying for these programs may require providing detailed medical documentation and undergoing a review process.

Healthcare coverage should also include access to a multidisciplinary team of specialists, including neurologists, respiratory therapists, and occupational therapists. Ensuring that your insurance covers these specialists can help provide comprehensive care tailored to the needs of ALS patients. Regularly reviewing and updating your healthcare coverage can help address changing medical needs and secure continued support.

WORKPLACE RIGHTS AND ACCOMMODATIONS

Workplace rights and accommodations are crucial for individuals with ALS who wish to continue working while managing their condition. The ADA provides protections for employees with disabilities, including the right to request reasonable accommodations to perform job duties. These accommodations may include modifications to the work environment, such as accessible workstations, flexible work hours, or assistive technologies.

Requesting accommodations involves communicating with your employer and providing documentation from healthcare professionals that outlines your needs. Employers are required by law to engage in an interactive process to determine appropriate accommodations. It is important to work collaboratively with your employer to find solutions that enable you to maintain your job while managing the effects of ALS.

Understanding your workplace rights also involves knowing how to address any potential discrimination or unfair treatment. If you encounter issues related to accommodations or workplace adjustments, documenting these instances and seeking assistance from human resources or legal counsel can help address and resolve these concerns. Being proactive and informed about your rights can help ensure a supportive and accommodating work environment.

ESTATE PLANNING AND ADVANCE DIRECTIVES

Estate planning and advance directives are essential components of managing ALS, as they address future healthcare decisions and the distribution of assets. Advance directives include documents such as living wills and durable powers of attorney that specify your preferences for medical treatment and appoint a trusted individual to make decisions on your behalf if you are unable to do so.

Creating an estate plan involves outlining how your assets will be distributed and identifying any guardianship arrangements for dependents. Working with an attorney who specializes in estate planning can help ensure that your wishes are clearly documented and legally binding. This process includes drafting wills, setting up trusts, and designating beneficiaries for financial accounts.

Advance directives should be reviewed and updated regularly to reflect any changes in your health status or preferences.

Sharing these documents with your healthcare providers, family members, and legal representatives ensures that your wishes are known and can be acted upon when needed. Proper planning and communication can provide peace of mind and ensure that your healthcare and financial decisions align with your goals.

CHAPTER NINE

SUPPORT SYSTEMS AND RESOURCES

SUPPORT GROUPS AND ORGANIZATIONS

Support groups and organizations play a crucial role in providing emotional and practical assistance for individuals with Amyotrophic Lateral Sclerosis (ALS) and their families. These groups offer a space where individuals can connect with others facing similar challenges, share experiences, and exchange practical advice on managing the disease. Many organizations, such as the ALS Association, provide resources for finding local support groups, which may include in-person meetings and online forums. These gatherings often facilitate peer support, allowing members to discuss coping strategies, treatment options, and daily living adjustments.

In addition to peer support, these organizations frequently offer various services such as educational materials, financial assistance programs, and access to specialized medical care. They may organize events like fundraisers and awareness campaigns, which not only support research but also help raise public understanding of ALS. Participation in these groups can be invaluable for both patients and their families, providing a sense of community and reducing feelings of isolation.

For those who are new to ALS or seeking guidance on available resources, contacting these organizations can be a beneficial first step. They often have dedicated staff who can provide information about local support networks and connect individuals with appropriate resources. Engaging with these groups can help families navigate the complexities of ALS while fostering a supportive environment.

ONLINE RESOURCES AND FORUMS

Online resources and forums offer a wealth of information and support for those affected by ALS. These platforms provide access to a broad range of resources, including medical research, treatment options, and patient testimonials. Websites dedicated to ALS often feature articles, videos, and webinars that cover various aspects of the disease, from diagnosis and treatment to managing symptoms and maintaining quality of life.

Forums and social media groups provide real-time support and a space for sharing experiences. These online communities allow individuals to connect with others worldwide, offering a platform for asking questions, sharing personal stories, and obtaining advice from both peers and experts. Participants can benefit from the collective knowledge and experiences of others who have navigated similar challenges.

Navigating online resources effectively requires understanding how to find credible information and engage with reputable communities. It's important to verify the credibility of sources and consult healthcare professionals when interpreting medical advice found online. Using these resources wisely can significantly enhance one's knowledge and support network.

PROFESSIONAL COUNSELING AND THERAPY

Professional counseling and therapy are essential for addressing the emotional and psychological impact of ALS. Psychologists, social workers, and therapists specializing in chronic illness can help patients and their families cope with the stress, anxiety, and emotional challenges associated with the disease. Therapy sessions provide a structured environment for discussing feelings, setting coping strategies, and managing the psychological burden of ALS.

Counselors can also assist with practical aspects of adjusting to life with ALS, such as navigating the healthcare system, planning for future care needs, and enhancing communication within the family. Therapeutic approaches may include individual therapy, family counseling, and cognitive-behavioral therapy, each tailored to address specific emotional or psychological issues.

For those seeking therapy, it's beneficial to consult healthcare providers for recommendations or search for licensed professionals with experience in chronic illness management. Regular sessions can offer ongoing support and help individuals and families adapt to the evolving challenges of ALS.

COMMUNITY AND CAREGIVER SUPPORT

Community support is vital for individuals with ALS and their caregivers. Local community programs often provide practical help such as respite care, transportation services, and assistance with daily tasks.

These resources can alleviate some of the burdens on caregivers, who often face significant physical and emotional strain while managing the needs of their loved ones.

Caregiver support groups offer a space for sharing experiences and strategies for managing caregiving responsibilities. These groups can help caregivers build a network of support, learn from others' experiences, and find practical advice for balancing caregiving with personal needs. Some communities also provide training sessions to equip caregivers with skills for the effective management of ALS symptoms.

Engaging with community resources and support services can make a significant difference in the quality of life for both patients and caregivers. It's important to explore local options and stay informed about available programs that can offer practical and emotional support.

EDUCATIONAL RESOURCES AND WORKSHOPS

Educational resources and workshops provide essential information and skills for managing ALS. These resources can include informational brochures, online courses, and hands-on workshops that cover various aspects of ALS, such as understanding the disease, managing symptoms, and adapting daily living activities. Workshops often offer practical demonstrations and interactive sessions, which can help patients and caregivers learn new techniques for managing the disease.

Specialized workshops may focus on topics such as physical therapy exercises, nutritional guidance, and adaptive technology, which can improve quality of life. These sessions are typically led by healthcare professionals or experts in ALS care, providing participants with up-to-date knowledge and practical skills.

To benefit from these educational opportunities, individuals should seek out reputable organizations and institutions that offer relevant programs. Staying informed and engaged with educational resources can empower patients and caregivers with the knowledge needed to navigate the complexities of ALS effectively.

CHAPTER TEN

DETAILED FAQS

WHAT ARE THE EARLY SYMPTOMS OF ALS?

Amyotrophic Lateral Sclerosis (ALS) begins with subtle symptoms that can be easily overlooked. Early signs often include muscle weakness or stiffness, which may first be noticeable in the hands, feet, or legs. This weakness can lead to difficulty with fine motor skills, such as buttoning a shirt or typing. Muscle cramps and twitching, known as fasciculations, are also common and might be mistaken for general fatigue or stress.

As the disease progresses, individuals may experience more pronounced difficulty with movement and coordination. For instance, walking may become awkward or unsteady, and tasks requiring physical dexterity can become challenging. Speech and swallowing difficulties may also develop, impacting daily activities and communication. Recognizing these early symptoms is crucial for timely intervention.

It's important to note that ALS symptoms can vary from person to person, and early signs may overlap with other neurological conditions. If you or someone you know begins to experience these symptoms, it's essential to consult a healthcare professional for a comprehensive evaluation and diagnosis.

HOW IS ALS DIAGNOSED AND WHAT TESTS ARE USED?

Diagnosing ALS involves a thorough medical evaluation to rule out other conditions that might mimic its symptoms. The diagnostic process typically begins with a detailed patient history and physical examination. Neurologists look for signs of muscle weakness, atrophy, and changes in reflexes, as well as any problems with speech, swallowing, or breathing.

Several tests are used to confirm an ALS diagnosis. Electromyography (EMG) measures the electrical activity in muscles, helping to identify abnormalities characteristic of ALS. Nerve conduction studies assess how well electrical signals travel along the nerves. In some cases, additional imaging tests such as MRI or CT scans may be used to rule out other conditions and to visualize the brain and spinal cord. A lumbar puncture (spinal tap) might also be performed to analyze cerebrospinal fluid for other possible causes of symptoms.

Since there is no single definitive test for ALS, the diagnosis is often based on a combination of clinical findings and test results. It is a process of exclusion, where other potential causes of the symptoms are ruled out, leading to a diagnosis of ALS.

WHAT TREATMENTS ARE CURRENTLY AVAILABLE FOR ALS?

Currently, there is no cure for ALS, but various treatments can help manage symptoms and improve quality of life. Medications such as Riluzole and Edaravone are approved to slow disease progression and may help prolong survival.

Riluzole is believed to reduce damage to motor neurons, while Edaravone is thought to have antioxidant properties that protect cells from oxidative stress.

Symptom management is a critical aspect of ALS treatment. Physical therapy can help maintain muscle strength and flexibility, while occupational therapy aids in adapting daily activities to the individual's abilities. Speech therapy is crucial for those experiencing difficulties with communication and swallowing. Additionally, nutritional support and respiratory care are important as the disease progresses, with interventions like feeding tubes or ventilators sometimes necessary.

Collaborative care from a multidisciplinary team, including neurologists, therapists, and support staff, is essential for the comprehensive management of ALS. These treatments and supportive measures aim to enhance comfort, maintain independence, and address specific needs as they arise.

HOW CAN I FIND SUPPORT GROUPS AND RESOURCES FOR ALS?

Finding support groups and resources for ALS can greatly benefit those affected by the disease. National organizations such as the ALS Association offer valuable information, support services, and opportunities to connect with others in similar situations. Their websites often provide directories of local chapters and support groups.

Online communities and forums are also valuable resources for connecting with others who have ALS or who are caregivers.

These platforms allow individuals to share experiences, advice, and emotional support. Additionally, local hospitals and clinics may have information on support groups and resources specific to your area.

Involving yourself in these communities can provide emotional support, practical advice, and a sense of connection with others facing similar challenges.

Engaging with these resources can help manage the impact of ALS on daily life and provide guidance on navigating the complexities of the disease.

WHAT ARE THE PROSPECTS FOR ALS RESEARCH AND TREATMENT?

Research into ALS is ongoing, with numerous studies exploring potential treatments and a cure. Advances in understanding the genetic and molecular mechanisms of ALS hold promise for developing targeted therapies. Researchers are investigating the role of gene mutations and how they contribute to the disease, with the hope of identifying new therapeutic targets.

Innovations in drug development and clinical trials are crucial for finding effective treatments. Therapies aimed at modifying disease progression or repairing damaged motor neurons are under investigation. Stem cell research and gene therapy are among the most promising areas, with the potential to offer new avenues for treatment.

The future of ALS research is hopeful, with increasing collaboration among scientists, clinicians, and advocacy organizations. Continued investment in research and clinical trials is essential for advancing our understanding of ALS and improving treatment options, ultimately aiming for a cure.